# WALL YOGA FOR SENIORS

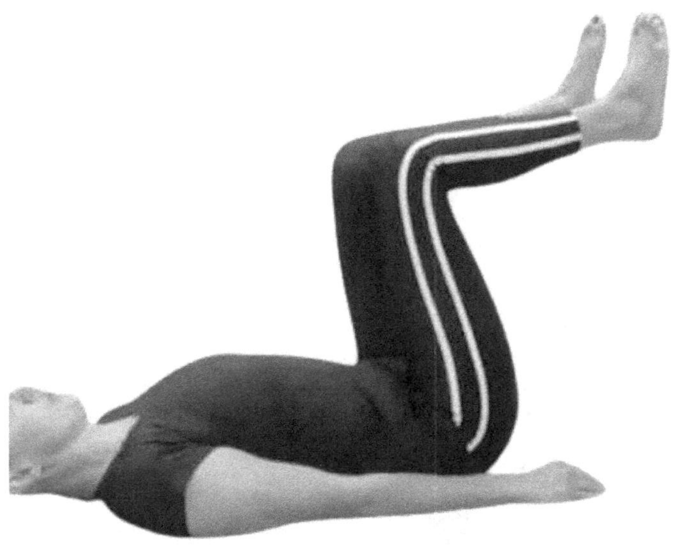

## 10 Minutes Low-Impact Exercises For Men And Women To Lose Weight And Enhance Mobility, Strength And Balance

Randy T. Lucas

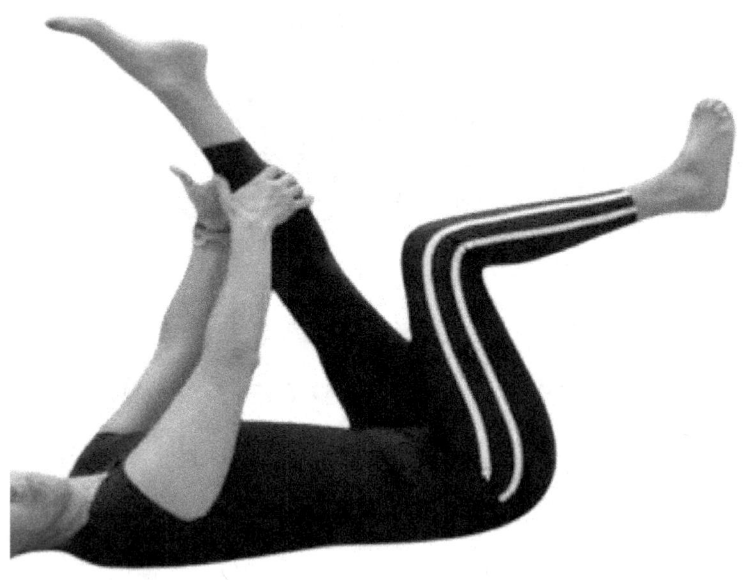

# Table of Contents

# INTRODUCTION

In a quiet corner of a bustling town, there lived a community of seniors who discovered a path to rejuvenation, vitality, and serenity through the practice of wall yoga. Among them was Tracy, a spirited 70-year-old who, until recently, felt the weight of age burdening her every movement. One fateful day, she stumbled upon a gentle yoga session tailored specifically for seniors, centered around the supportive embrace of a wall.

At first tentative, Tracy soon found herself drawn into the world of wall yoga. With each stretch against the sturdy surface, she felt a surge of newfound energy coursing through her body. The wall became her steady companion, offering support as she ventured into poses she once thought were out of reach. Through regular practice, she discovered a sense of freedom in movement she hadn't felt in years.

Like Tracy, many seniors around the globe are seeking ways to maintain an active lifestyle while respecting the changes their bodies undergo. Wall yoga emerged as a beacon of hope, offering a gentle yet effective means to address the unique needs of aging bodies. This guide seeks to unveil the transformative potential of wall yoga, tailored specifically to the cherished seniors seeking solace, strength, and renewed vitality.

In the following chapters, we embark on a journey designed to unlock the manifold benefits of wall yoga for seniors. We delve into its profound impact on relaxation, mobility, strength, posture, and overall well-being. With an emphasis on safety and customization, this guide aims to provide a sanctuary for seniors to explore and harness the healing powers of wall yoga.

As we venture forward, let this guide serve not just as a manual but as a companion on your path toward a more vibrant, balanced, and joyful life. Together, let us embrace the wall as a symbol of support, resilience, and transformation, as we discover the incredible journey that wall yoga offers to the heart, body, and soul of every senior practitioner.

# CHAPTER 1

## Understanding Wall Yoga for Seniors

Wall yoga for seniors is a specialized practice that merges the principles of traditional yoga with the support of a wall. This unique approach caters specifically to the needs of older adults, providing a safe and effective way to experience the benefits of yoga.

The primary focus of wall yoga for seniors is to use the wall as a prop for support, stability, and alignment. The wall acts as a steady companion, offering a sense of security while allowing practitioners to explore yoga poses with greater ease and comfort. It becomes an anchor, enabling seniors to deepen their stretches, maintain balance, and engage in movements that might otherwise be challenging due to physical limitations or reduced mobility.

This form of yoga emphasizes gentle movements, mindful breathing, and poses that are easily modifiable to accommodate individual abilities and limitations. By utilizing the wall as a stabilizing force, seniors can gradually build strength, improve flexibility, enhance posture, and promote relaxation.

One of the beauties of wall yoga for seniors is its adaptability. Poses can be modified by adjusting the distance from the wall or by using props such as yoga blocks or straps to ensure comfort and safety. Additionally, the practice can be tailored to address specific concerns, such as joint stiffness, balance issues, or chronic conditions commonly experienced in older age.

Moreover, wall yoga for seniors fosters a supportive and inclusive environment. It encourages a sense of community, allowing individuals to embark on their yoga journey at their own pace while fostering connections with others in a similar phase of life.

In essence, wall yoga for seniors is not just about physical exercise; it's a holistic approach to well-being. It honors the unique needs of aging bodies, offering a gentle yet powerful means for seniors to enhance their overall health, flexibility, and emotional balance through the guidance and support of a wall.

# Benefits of Wall Yoga for Senior Practitioners

**1. Enhanced Stability:** The wall provides a stable support system, aiding seniors in maintaining balance during yoga poses, reducing the risk of falls, and building confidence in movement.

**2. Improved Flexibility:** Using the wall as a prop allows seniors to safely deepen stretches, gradually increasing flexibility in muscles and joints, leading to increased range of motion.

**3. Gentle Strength Building:** Wall yoga incorporates poses that engage various muscle groups, promoting gentle strength development without straining joints or muscles excessively.

**4. Better Posture Alignment:** With the aid of the wall, seniors can work on aligning their bodies properly, correcting posture imbalances, and reducing discomfort associated with poor posture.

**5. Joint Mobility:** Wall yoga encourages gentle movement of joints, improving mobility and reducing stiffness, particularly beneficial for seniors dealing with arthritis or joint-related issues.

**6. Stress Reduction:** Practicing yoga against the wall encourages relaxation through controlled breathing and mindful movements, aiding in stress reduction and promoting a sense of calmness.

**7. Increased Body Awareness:** The wall acts as a tactile guide, helping seniors become more aware of their body's position in space, fostering mindfulness and a deeper mind-body connection.

**8. Safe and Accessible Practice:** Wall yoga offers a safe and accessible way for seniors to participate in yoga, accommodating different physical abilities and allowing for modifications as needed.

**9. Support for Chronic Conditions:** It can be adapted to support seniors dealing with chronic health conditions such as osteoporosis, hypertension, or arthritis, offering gentle therapeutic benefits.

**10. Community and Social Engagement:** Participating in wall yoga classes fosters a sense of community among seniors, providing an opportunity for social interaction and support, contributing to overall well-being.

# Safety Precautions and Considerations

**1. Consultation with a Healthcare Professional:** Before starting any new exercise regimen, especially for seniors with pre-existing health conditions, it's advisable to consult a healthcare professional to ensure yoga is safe and suitable.

**2. Warm-Up Routine:** Begin with gentle warm-up exercises to prepare the body for yoga practice, gradually increasing intensity to avoid strain or injury.

**3. Proper Wall Distance:** Maintain an appropriate distance from the wall during poses to prevent overextension or strain on muscles and joints.

**4. Mindful Movements:** Practice mindfulness during movements, moving slowly and with control, avoiding sudden or jerky motions that could lead to injury.

**5. Use of Props:** Utilize yoga props such as blocks or straps to modify poses and provide additional support, especially for seniors with limited flexibility or mobility.

**6. Awareness of Body Signals:** Pay attention to your body's signals. If a pose causes pain or discomfort beyond mild stretching sensations, ease out of it or modify the pose.

**7. Breathing Awareness:** Focus on steady and controlled breathing throughout the practice to enhance relaxation and avoid breath-holding, which can increase blood pressure.

**8. Avoid Overexertion:** Seniors should avoid pushing themselves too hard. Listen to your body and take breaks whenever needed, not striving for perfection in poses.

**9. Adaptation and Modification:** Modify poses according to individual abilities and limitations, ensuring safety and comfort while still gaining benefits from the practice.

**10. Hydration and Rest:** Stay hydrated before, during, and after the practice. Adequate rest between poses and after the session is crucial for recovery and injury prevention.

These safety precautions and considerations aim to create a safe and nurturing environment for seniors engaging in wall yoga, allowing them to reap the benefits of the practice while minimizing the risk of injury or discomfort.

# CHAPTER 2

# Relaxation and Stress Relief

## Gentle Wall Stretches to Relax the Body:

**Wall Supported Forward Fold:**

- Stand facing the wall a few feet away.

- Lean forward, placing palms or forearms on the wall at shoulder height.

- Relax head and neck, feeling a gentle stretch along the back and hamstrings.

**Wall Chest Opener:**

- Stand beside the wall, extending one arm sideways at shoulder height.

- Turn body away from the wall, feeling a gentle stretch across the chest and shoulder.

- Hold, then switch sides to stretch the other side.

**Legs-Up-the-Wall Pose (Viparita Karani):**

- Sit close to the wall and lie down on your back.

- Extend legs up against the wall, relaxing arms by your sides.

- Stay in this position to promote relaxation and ease tension in the legs.

# Breathing Techniques for Relaxation and Calmness:

**Wall-Supported Belly Breathing:**

- Sit comfortably against the wall with knees bent.

- Place one hand on the chest and the other on the belly.

- Inhale deeply through the nose, feeling the belly rise; exhale slowly, feeling it fall.

**Alternate Nostril Breathing (Nadi Shodhana):**

- Sit comfortably against the wall.

- Use thumb to close one nostril, inhale through the open nostril, then switch and exhale through the other.

- Repeat, alternating nostrils, focusing on rhythmic breathing.

**4-7-8 Breathing:**

- Sit comfortably with your back against the wall.

- Inhale deeply for a count of 4, hold for 7, exhale slowly for 8 counts.

- Repeat this pattern for several cycles to induce relaxation.

# Guided Meditation Practices Against the Wall:

**Wall-Supported Body Scan Meditation:**

- Sit or lie comfortably against the wall.

- Close eyes and bring attention to different body parts, releasing tension gradually from toes to head.

**Wall Gazing Meditation:**

- Sit comfortably close to the wall.
- Soften gaze and focus on a spot or object on the wall, observing thoughts as they come and go.

**Mantra Meditation Against the Wall:**

- Sit comfortably against the wall with eyes closed.
- Silently repeat a calming mantra with each breath, allowing it to guide your meditation practice.

These exercises, when practiced against the wall, aim to promote relaxation, calmness, and stress reduction for seniors engaging in wall yoga.

# CHAPTER 3

# Mobility and Flexibility

## Wall-Assisted Stretches for Improved Flexibility:

**Wall Supported Hamstring Stretch:**

- Place one foot at hip height on the wall while standing with your back to it.

- Lean forward, keeping your back straight, feeling a stretch in the back of the leg.

- Hold for a few breaths, then switch legs.

**Wall Pectoral Stretch:**

- Stand with one arm extended on the wall at shoulder height.

- Gently turn your body away from the wall, feeling a stretch across the chest and front of the shoulder.

- Hold, then switch sides.

# Wall Supported Quadriceps Stretch:

- Stand facing away from the wall, holding onto it for support.

- Bend one knee, bringing your foot toward your buttocks, feeling a stretch in the front of the thigh.

- Hold onto the wall for balance, then switch legs.

# Joint Mobility Exercises Using the Wall:

**Wall Shoulder Circles:**

- Stand facing the wall with arms extended at shoulder height.

- Slowly make circular motions with your arms against the wall, gently mobilizing the shoulder joints.

- Reverse the direction of the circles after a few repetitions.

**Wall Ankle Alphabet:**

- Sit on the floor with your back against the wall, legs extended.

-Raise up one leg and draw the alphabet with your toes against the wall, working on ankle mobility and flexibility.

- Switch legs and repeat the exercise.

**Wall Hip Flexor Stretch:**

- Kneel down facing the wall, with one knee close to the wall and the other knee on the ground.

- Lean forward, keeping your back straight, feeling a stretch in the front of the hip and thigh.

- Hold, then switch sides.

**Enhancing Range of Motion with Wall Support:**

- Wall-Assisted Squats:

- Stand with your back against the wall and feet shoulder-width apart.

- Slide down into a squatting position, using the wall for support and stability.

- Hold for a few seconds, then return to standing.

**Wall Calf Stretch:**

- Stand facing the wall with one foot back, heel on the ground.

- Lean forward, keeping the back leg straight, feeling a stretch in the calf.

- Hold, then switch legs.

**Wall Supported Backbend Stretch:**

- Stand facing the wall, a couple of feet away.

- Lean backward, placing your hands on the wall for support, feeling a gentle stretch in the front of the body.

- Hold the position, then return to standing.

# CHAPTER 4

# Strength and Balance

## Building Strength through Wall-Supported Poses:

**Wall-Supported Warrior Pose:**

- Stand sideways to the wall with one hand resting lightly against it.
- Step the outer leg back into a lunge position, bending the front knee while keeping the back leg straight.
- Hold the pose, feeling the engagement in the legs and core, then switch sides.

**Wall-Supported Chair Pose:**

- Stand with your back against the wall and lower into a squat position, as if sitting in an imaginary chair.

- Press your back into the wall for support and hold the pose, engaging thighs and core muscles.

**Wall-Supported Tree Pose:**

- Stand beside the wall and place the sole of one foot against the inner thigh or calf of the opposite leg.
- Use the wall for balance support as you bring your palms together in front of your chest.
- Hold the pose, focusing on balance and stability, then switch sides.

# Balancing Poses Utilizing the Wall for Stability:

**Wall-Assisted Leg Lifts:**

- Stand facing the wall with hands resting lightly against it for support.
- Lift one leg to the side or to the back, maintaining balance with the support of the wall.
- Lower the leg and switch sides.

**Wall-Supported Warrior III Pose:**

- Stand facing away from the wall and extend one leg straight behind you.
- Lean forward, reaching arms forward, and rest hands against the wall for balance.
- Hold the pose, aiming for a straight line from head to extended heel, then switch sides.

**Wall Plank Pose:**

- Face the wall and place hands on the wall, shoulder-width apart, in a push-up position.
- Straighten your body, engaging core muscles, forming a plank position with feet hip-width apart.
- Hold the pose, focusing on stability and alignment.

# Core Strengthening Exercises Against the Wall:

**Wall Sit with Twist:**

  - Sit against the wall in a squat position.

  - Lift one foot off the ground and twist your torso to touch the lifted knee with the opposite elbow.

  - Return to center and switch sides, engaging the core muscles throughout.

**Wall Crunches:**

  - Lie down facing the wall, with legs raised and feet against the wall.

  - Perform crunches, lifting your upper body towards the wall, engaging the abdominal muscles.

**Leg Raises against the Wall:**

  - Lie down facing the wall with legs extended upward against the wall.

  - Lift legs up and down, engaging the lower abdominal muscles, maintaining control and stability.

# CHAPTER 5

# Posture and Alignment

## Correcting Posture with Wall Alignment Techniques:

**Wall Standing Posture Check:**

- Stand against the wall with heels, buttocks, shoulders, and back of the head touching it.
- Ensure natural curves of the spine by slightly tucking chin, engaging core muscles, and relaxing shoulders down.

**Wall Shoulder Blade Squeeze:**

- Stand with your back against the wall, arms by your sides.
- Gently squeeze your shoulder blades together, holding for a few seconds, then release.

**Wall Forward Head Posture Correction:**

- Stand with your back against the wall.

- Gently press the back of your head against the wall, tucking your chin slightly to align the head with the spine.

# Wall-Supported Spine Strengthening Exercises:

**Wall Cat-Cow Stretch:**

- Stand facing the wall, placing hands on the wall at shoulder height.

- Perform a cat-cow stretch by arching and rounding the spine, feeling the movement along the entire length of the spine.

**Wall Cobra Pose:**

- Lie on your stomach, facing away from the wall, with palms on the wall at shoulder height.

- Press into the wall, lifting your chest and head while engaging the back muscles, holding the pose.

**Wall Supported Bridge Pose:**

- Lie on your back facing the wall, knees bent, and feet flat against the wall.
- Lift your hips off the ground, pressing into the wall for support, engaging glutes and core muscles.

# Improving Body Awareness and Alignment:

**Wall-Assisted Standing Balance:**

- Stand sideways to the wall, lightly placing fingertips on it for support.
- Lift one leg off the ground and find your balance, focusing on body alignment, then switch sides.

**Wall Proprioception Exercise:**

- Stand facing the wall, gently close your eyes.
- Slowly lift one foot off the ground and hold, focusing on maintaining balance and body awareness without visual cues from the wall.

**Wall Squat with Alignment Check:**

- Stand against the wall and perform a squat, sliding down with back against the wall.
- Hold the squat position, checking knee alignment over ankles and maintaining a neutral spine against the wall.

# CHAPTER 6

# Wall Yoga Sequences

## Beginner Wall Yoga Sequence for Seniors:

**Wall Supported Mountain Pose:**

- Stand with feet hip-width apart, back against the wall.
- Relax shoulders, engage core, and feel the support of the wall. Hold for 5 breaths.

**Wall Supported Forward Fold:**

- Stand a few feet away from the wall.
- Lean forward, placing hands or forearms on the wall for support. Hold for 3-5 breaths.

**Wall Cobra Pose:**

- Lie on your stomach, facing away from the wall.
- Place palms on the wall at shoulder height, lift chest, and hold for 3-4 breaths.

**Wall Assisted Chair Pose:**

- Stand with back against the wall, lower into a squat position.
- Use the wall for support, engaging thighs and core. Hold for 4-5 breaths.

**Wall-Supported Child's Pose:**

- Kneel in front of the wall, gently rest forehead and arms on the wall.
- Relax into the pose, focusing on steady breaths. Hold for 5-6 breaths.

# Intermediate Wall Yoga Sequence for Progression:

**Wall Supported Warrior II Pose:**

- Stand sideways to the wall, extend arms at shoulder height.

- Bend front knee, feeling the support of the wall. Hold for 4-5 breaths on each side.

**Wall Side Plank Pose:**

- Place one hand on the wall at shoulder height.

- Stack feet and hips, lifting into a side plank position. Hold for 4-5 breaths on each side.

**Wall Assisted Downward Dog:**

- Face away from the wall, place hands on the wall at hip height.

- Walk feet back, creating an inverted V shape. Hold for 3-4 breaths.

**Wall Supported Boat Pose:**

- Sit on the floor facing the wall, legs extended.
- Lift legs, creating a V shape, lean back and place hands on the wall for support. Hold for 4-5 breaths.

**Wall Supported Pigeon Pose:**

- Sit sideways to the wall, place one leg against the wall.
- Gently lean forward, feeling a hip stretch. Hold for 4-5 breaths on each side.

# Advanced Wall Yoga Flow for Increased Challenge:

**Wall Supported Headstand Preparation:**


- Place forearms on the ground a few inches from the wall.

- Lift hips into a dolphin pose, engaging core muscles. Hold for 3-4 breaths.


**Wall Supported Handstand Preparation:**


- Stand facing the wall, place hands on the ground shoulder-width apart.

- Lift one leg, then the other, into a handstand prep position, using the wall for support. Hold for 3-4 breaths.


**Wall Assisted Wheel Pose:**


- Lie on your back facing the wall, bend knees, place feet on the wall.

- Lift hips, walk hands towards feet, and press into the wall for a supported backbend. Hold for 4-5 breaths.

**Wall Supported Extended Side Angle Pose:**

- Stand sideways to the wall, feet wide apart.

- Bend one knee, place elbow on the knee, and extend the other arm overhead against the wall. Hold for 4-5 breaths on each side.

**Wall Supported Revolved Triangle Pose:**

- Stand facing the wall, step one foot back and place the hand on the wall.

- Twist the torso and extend the opposite arm toward the ceiling. Hold for 4-5 breaths on each side.

These sequences cater to different levels of expertise, utilizing the wall for support and gradually increasing the challenge for seniors practicing wall yoga.

# CHAPTER 7

# Special Considerations and Modifications

## Adapting Wall Yoga Poses for Seniors with Physical Limitations

**Reduced Range of Motion:**

- Use props like straps or blocks to accommodate limited flexibility.
- Opt for partial or modified poses, adjusting according to individual comfort levels.

**Balance Challenges:**

- Perform poses near a wall or chair for extra support and stability.

- Focus on engaging core muscles to enhance balance during poses.

**Joint Sensitivity:**

- Practice gentle movements and avoid extreme joint angles.
- Perform smaller movements or use the wall for light support to reduce joint strain.

**Limited Mobility:**

- Modify standing poses by using the wall for balance or opting for seated variations.
- Incorporate chair yoga poses or practice in a seated position against the wall.

# Modifying Wall Yoga for Specific Health Conditions:

## 1. Arthritis:

- Choose gentle movements that don't exacerbate joint pain.

- Use the wall for support during stretches, allowing for modifications to accommodate sensitive joints.

## 2. Osteoporosis:

- Avoid forward-bending poses that strain the spine.

- Emphasize gentle backbends and standing poses for strength without compression on the spine.

## 3. Hypertension:

- Focus on slow, controlled breathing techniques.

- Avoid inversions or poses that put excessive pressure on the head or neck.

## 4. Back Pain:

- Perform supported backbends against the wall to alleviate pressure on the spine.

- Engage in gentle twists and stretches to promote flexibility and alleviate tension.

## 5. Balance Disorders:

- Practice poses close to a wall or with a chair for added stability.

- Concentrate on grounding and stability while engaging in standing poses.

## 6. Respiratory Conditions:

- Incorporate breathing exercises in a seated or reclined position against the wall.

- Focus on controlled, deep breathing to improve lung capacity without causing strain.

# CONCLUSION

As we bring our exploration of Wall Yoga for Seniors to a close, it's evident that this practice is nothing short of a transformative journey toward holistic well-being. It's more than just about touching the wall or holding a pose; it's about discovering a newfound sense of vitality, balance, and harmony.

Amidst the serenity of the yoga space, the wall becomes an ally, a trusted support that facilitates deeper stretches, ensures stability, and encourages a sense of exploration. It's akin to a gentle guide, gently nudging seniors to delve deeper into their physical capabilities while fostering a profound connection between mind and body.

Through the serene stretches, intentional breathwork, and the gentle embrace of the wall, seniors unlock a sanctuary where every movement feels purposeful and every moment becomes an opportunity for self-discovery. It's within these moments that the wall becomes more than just a prop; it becomes a conduit to unlock hidden strengths, enhance flexibility, and promote a deeper sense of self-awareness.

Yet, beyond the physical benefits, Wall Yoga for Seniors resonates as a gateway to mental rejuvenation and emotional tranquility. It's a practice that transcends age, offering a haven for seniors to unwind, release tension, and find solace amidst life's hustle and bustle.

This journey through Wall Yoga is a testament to resilience, adaptability, and the sheer vibrancy that defines the golden years. It's an invitation for seniors to embrace the beauty of movement, to foster a supple body, a tranquil mind, and a rejuvenated spirit.

So, as we bid adieu to this exploration, let the wall stand as a symbol of unwavering support, resilience, and endless opportunities for seniors to relish each stretch, savor every breath, and revel in the vibrant experience of Wall Yoga—an oasis of wellness, vitality, and grace in the journey of graceful aging.

# FITNESS

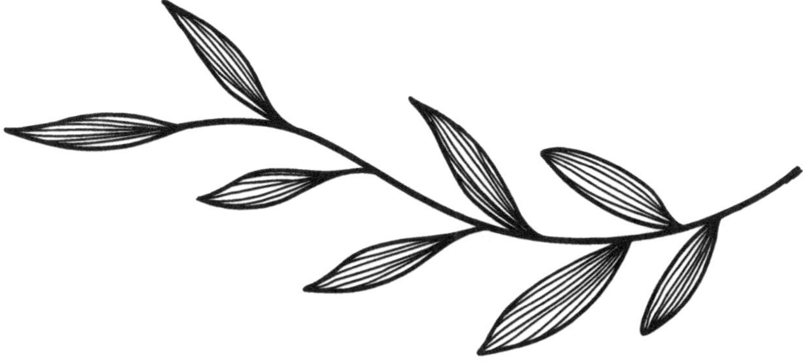

# PLANNER

# Fitness Planner

**NAME:**                 **DATE:**

## BREAKFAST

## LUNCH

## DINNER

## SNACK

| EXERCISE | SET | REP | NOTES |
|----------|-----|-----|-------|
|          |     |     |       |

# Fitness Planner

**NAME:**  **DATE:**

## BREAKFAST

## LUNCH

## DINNER

## SNACK

## EXERCISE

## SET   REP   NOTES

# Fitness
# Planner

**NAME:**     **DATE:**

### BREAKFAST

### LUNCH

### DINNER

### SNACK

### EXERCISE     SET     REP     NOTES

# Fitness
# Planner

**NAME:**                    **DATE:**

## BREAKFAST

## LUNCH

## DINNER

## SNACK

## EXERCISE          SET        REP        NOTES

# Fitness Planner

**NAME:**                    **DATE:**

### BREAKFAST                 LUNCH

### DINNER                    SNACK

### EXERCISE          SET     REP     NOTES

# Fitness Planner

**NAME:**                    **DATE:**

## BREAKFAST

## LUNCH

## DINNER

## SNACK

## EXERCISE          SET       REP       NOTES

# Fitness Planner

NAME:                    DATE:

BREAKFAST                LUNCH

DINNER                   SNACK

EXERCISE        SET      REP      NOTES

# Fitness Planner

**NAME:**            **DATE:**

## BREAKFAST

## LUNCH

## DINNER

## SNACK

| EXERCISE | SET | REP | NOTES |
| --- | --- | --- | --- |
|  |  |  |  |

# Fitness Planner

**NAME:**

**DATE:**

## BREAKFAST

## LUNCH

## DINNER

## SNACK

## EXERCISE

SET

REP

NOTES

# Fitness Planner

**NAME:**       **DATE:**

## BREAKFAST

## LUNCH

## DINNER

## SNACK

## EXERCISE

| SET | REP | NOTES |
| --- | --- | --- |
|  |  |  |